Génesis Andrea Bolívar Parada
Angélica Del Valle Mujica Medina

Seroprevalence of infectious diseases

Génesis Andrea Bolívar Parada
Angélica Del Valle Mujica Medina

Seroprevalence of infectious diseases

of blood transmission in blood bank donors at Coromoto Hospital: July 2019-July 2020

Imprint

Any brand names and product names mentioned in this book are subject to trademark, brand or patent protection and are trademarks or registered trademarks of their respective holders. The use of brand names, product names, common names, trade names, product descriptions etc. even without a particular marking in this work is in no way to be construed to mean that such names may be regarded as unrestricted in respect of trademark and brand protection legislation and could thus be used by anyone.

Cover image: www.ingimage.com

This book is a translation from the original published under ISBN 978-613-9-40663-0.

Publisher:
Sciencia Scripts
is a trademark of
Dodo Books Indian Ocean Ltd. and OmniScriptum S.R.L publishing group

120 High Road, East Finchley, London, N2 9ED, United Kingdom
Str. Armeneasca 28/1, office 1, Chisinau MD-2012, Republic of Moldova, Europe
Printed at: see last page
ISBN: 978-620-7-98112-0

ACKNOWLEDGMENTS

We thank God for giving us life and allowing us to reach this point in our academic formation.

To our parents, whose unconditional support, patience and love have led us to be the people we are today, and who constantly motivated us to reach this achievement.

To our loved ones, family and friends, who in many ways were present along the way, always helping to lighten the load.

To our tutors, collaborators during this process, who, with their guidance, knowledge, and teachings, allowed the development of this work.

To the Military Academy of Medicine, for welcoming us into its scientific bosom, and allowing us to acquire the knowledge to train as Military Surgeons of excellence.

To the Coromoto Hospital of Maracaibo, especially to the Blood Bank, and to all the professionals who opened their doors to us with the best disposition and helped us to complete this project.

Without all of you, it would not have been possible.

DEDICATION

To God, for allowing us to successfully complete our career, and for the strength in every moment.

To our parents, with much love and affection, we dedicate all the effort and commitment put into the realization of this work.

To us, as thesis partners, for our effort, dedication, perseverance, and mutual support in every ups and downs during this career.

SUMMARY

The transfusion of blood or its derivatives has become an essential part for public health providers and, therefore, for blood banks. For this reason, it is currently stipulated that screening tests of blood units are mandatory for the detection of agents potentially transmissible through transfusions, which can cause diseases if not identified in a timely manner. The present research is a retrospective, cross-sectional, non-experimental, descriptive, descriptive study, whose total population consisted of voluntary donor users who attended the Blood Bank of the Coromoto Hospital of Maracaibo in the period July 2019-July 2020, and who met the inclusion and exclusion criteria of the study. A total of 3846 patients were evaluated, of which 128 were positive (3.32%) for any of the serological tests performed in this institution; likewise, 63 serologies corresponded to Syphilis (49.2%), obtaining the highest number of cases; 53 samples for anti-HBc (41.4%); 6 to HIV (4.7%); 4 cases with HbsAg (3.1%); 3 serologies for both Chagas and HCV (2.3%); and finally HTLV-1 with 1 case (0.8%).

Key words: *transfusion, blood bank, donor, serological tests, syphilis.*

E-mail: angelicamujica7@gmail.com/genesisbolivar10@gmail.com

Table of Contents

CHAPTER 1: THE PROBLEM

PROBLEM STATEMENT

Human blood is the only source of erythrocytes, platelets, plasma, and also includes coagulation factors. Transfusion is known as the simplest form of organ transplantation as it is transferred from a donor to a patient to temporarily correct a deficiency or impairment of a function[1] .

As this is a transplant process, it is important to perform prophylactic tests on both the donor and the recipient to ensure compatibility between them and especially to rule out infectious processes that can be transmitted through blood transfusions and blood derivatives[2] .

It is because of this that the health centers opted for the creation of the well-known blood banks, which are entities in charge of the regulation of these blood products, including the rigorous selection process of donors and the specific screening tests used to confirm the safe reception and use of the blood.

For this reason, blood transfusion or its derivatives has become an essential part for public health providers and, therefore, for blood banks; mainly due to the increase in accidents and medical needs, which are some of the elements that have led to the growing demand for blood.

In this regard, it is currently stipulated that blood units must undergo mandatory screening tests for the detection of agents potentially transmissible through transfusions, which can cause diseases if not identified in a timely manner; some of them are: antibodies for the human immunodeficiency virus (HIV); antibodies for hepatitis C; surface antigens for hepatitis B (HbAgS); serology for syphilis, among others[3] .

Thus, it is important to know that transmission of infectious agents through blood transfusion can occur for four reasons. The first is the collection of blood during the window period, defined as the period during which the donor is infected with a virus, but shows no signs or symptoms and the results of serological tests are negative; for human immunodeficiency virus (HIV) and hepatitis B virus (HBV), at least 90% of the risk is attributable to the window period, while for hepatitis C virus (HCV) it is 73 to 88%. The second is the existence of asymptomatic donors, chronic carriers of a transmissible infection, with persistently negative laboratory test results. The third is due to infections with mutants or strains undetectable by tests. Finally, technical errors in the laboratory; this last factor is important because it is human-dependent and should therefore be the subject of constant concern in view of the increase in automation; it is avoided by the consistent application of a quality assurance policy. For human error to be of clinical significance, a seropositive specimen must be reported as non-reactive (false negative)[4] .

In view of the above, it is understood that the transmission of infectious pathologies through transfusions constitutes one of the most serious threats to public health, so that blood should be subjected to a precise process of study to ensure the stability of its quality, and serological studies should be systematically performed. There are still restrictions that increase the risk components of seropositive individuals due to the high frequency of transfusions, thus constituting a primary means of transmission.

One of the viruses transmitted by contact with body fluids is the hepatitis B virus, which could be positive or negative for surface antigen (HBsAg); although, due to screening programs, its transmission by transfusion has decreased significantly[5] .

On the other hand, transfusions are the cause of a large number of cases of hepatitis C, an important public health problem on the planet, since well over half of the people who remain in contact with it develop chronic hepatitis, later leading to liver cirrhosis and the development of hepatocellular carcinoma, the greatest effect of the same. Likewise, intravenous drug use, tattooing, occupational hazard and heterosexual promiscuous behavior are also among the hazard components. It has likewise been predetermined that minimizing the number of transfusions decreases the danger of hepatitis C virus infection[6] .

Another disease of infectious origin is Acquired

Immunodeficiency Syndrome (AIDS); however, since 1985, with the discovery that HIV could be transmitted through blood transfusions, health authorities focused their attention on detection in laboratories and blood banks, considerably reducing post-transfusion transmission[7].

In addition, HTLV-I (human T-cell lymphotropic virus type 1) can be pointed out as one of the infectious agents capable of being transmitted through the transfusion route. It is essential to know that 90% of those who carry this virus can remain asymptomatic; however, the other 10% have the capacity to develop diseases that can be very severe, such as lymphoma and adult T-cell leukemia[8].

Similarly, syphilis is included as an infectious, endemic, chronic disease, with asymptomatic periods, caused by *Treponema pallidum,* a highly infectious mobile spirochete. Although sexual contact is the most common form of transmission, antibody testing for this disease is also required before transfusion, since transmission of this microorganism is possible through the administration of blood or its derivatives; however, it is a rare complication when blood preserved for more than 72 hours is used, since it has been shown that *T. pallidum* does not survive refrigerator temperature beyond that time. In contrast, the danger of syphilis transmission exists when freshly drawn blood is transfused[9].

Thus, Chagas disease also represents a serious public health problem in many Latin American countries. The causative parasite is *Trypanosoma cruzi,* a flagellated protozoan. The disease is transmitted through the feces of insect vectors, bedbugs of the species *Triatoma maculata* and *Rhodnius prolixus*, the latter being the most common in Venezuela, commonly known as "pito". The second source of transmission is blood transfusions, where all blood components are infectious[10].

For this reason, it is considered essential to know the studies carried out on the epidemiology of these infections in the blood donor population, which in some way can be a reflection of the epidemiological behavior in the general population.

For all the above mentioned, it is unquestionable the responsibility that blood banks have; health agencies that must ensure a blood product that provides benefits for both the recipient and the donor. That is why the Coromoto Hospital, located in the Maracaibo municipality of Zulia State, has a Blood Bank that covers the demand of all the medical services available (General Surgery, Caumatology, Intensive Care, Internal Medicine, Pediatrics, Gynecology and Obstetrics, Hematology, Oncology and Nephrology, among others), where a large percentage of patients require blood transfusions and/or its derivatives. This hospital has an area of influence of more than one million inhabitants, serving more than 4 thousand blood donors per year. For this reason, this research will be carried out in order to determine the prevalence of seropositivity for blood-borne infectious diseases in donors of the Blood Bank of the Coromoto Hospital in Maracaibo-Venezuela, attended from July 2019 to July 2020.

PROBLEM FORMULATION

Having stated the problem regarding the object of study, the formulation of the problem is based on the following questions:

What is the seroprevalence of blood-borne infectious diseases in blood bank donors of the Coromoto Hospital of Maracaibo-Venezuela, in the period 2019-2020?

What is the most prevalent blood-borne infectious disease in blood bank donors of the Coromoto Hospital of Maracaibo-Venezuela, in the period 2019-2020?

What is the seroprevalence of blood-borne infectious diseases in blood bank donors of the Coromoto Hospital of Maracaibo-Venezuela, in the period 2019-2020 according to sex?

What is the seroprevalence of blood-borne infectious diseases in blood bank donors of the Coromoto Hospital of Maracaibo-Venezuela, in the period 2019-2020 according to age groups?

What is the seroprevalence of blood-borne infectious diseases in blood bank donors of the Coromoto Hospital of Maracaibo-

Venezuela, in the period 2019-2020 according to origin?

RESEARCH OBJECTIVES

GENERAL OBJECTIVE

✓ To determine the seroprevalence of blood-borne infectious diseases in blood bank donors of the Coromoto Hospital of Maracaibo-Venezuela, in the period 2019-2020.

SPECIFIC OBJECTIVES

1. To determine the frequency of each of the blood-borne diseases in donors of the blood bank of the Coromoto Hospital of Maracaibo-Venezuela, in the period 2019-2020.
2. To determine the seroprevalence of blood-borne infectious diseases in blood bank donors of the Coromoto Hospital of Maracaibo-Venezuela, in the period 2019-2020 according to sex.
3. To know the seroprevalence of blood-borne infectious diseases in blood bank donors of the Coromoto Hospital of Maracaibo-Venezuela, in the period 2019-2020 according to age groups and most frequent precedence.
4. To establish the relationship between blood-borne infectious diseases in blood bank donors of the Coromoto Hospital of Maracaibo-Venezuela, in the period 2019-2020 and their sociodemographic variables.

JUSTIFICATION

As is well known, blood transfusions have become an essential part for public health service providers and blood banks in general, since the increase in accidents and medical needs are some of the elements that have led to the growing demand for blood products.

Currently, mandatory screening of blood units is stipulated for the detection of potentially transfusion-transmissible agents such as: antibodies for human immunodeficiency virus (HIV); antibodies for hepatitis C; hepatitis B surface antigens (HbAgS); serology for syphilis, and Chagas disease, among others. However, careful attention to the immunologic and infectious problems of blood transfusion reduces the risks inherent in them, but cannot eliminate them entirely.

Therefore, the importance of knowing the seroprevalence of infectious markers in the donor population should be taken into account, since this is to avoid the use of unsafe blood, and as far as possible, to have safe blood products to be used and dispatched to the different services provided by the Hospital to the affiliates and their families. Given this reality, the present research will expose the seroprevalence of blood-borne infectious diseases in donors who came to the blood bank of the Coromoto Hospital of Maracaibo Venezuela, during the period 2019-2020; in addition, the identification of infectious markers will allow knowing which blood-borne disease prevails more frequently in this population.

Likewise, the proposed research will contribute to demonstrate the quality of serological screening based on the detection of infectious agents. Likewise, the results of the study will help to create epidemiological surveillance plans in the affected population, as well as to know the frequency of new positive cases related to sex, age and origin, thus improving the criteria for the acceptance of donors and, therefore, decreasing the risk of transmission of the infectious agents indicated above in this population.

On the other hand, this information could be used by the directors of the Coromoto Hospital for decision making in order to improve the services provided by this care center, as well as to manage with governmental and non-governmental organizations; in order to raise awareness in society on issues related to voluntary donation and risky sexual relations. The data analyzed should also serve as a point of reference and as an incentive for future research by students of related careers, health personnel interested in the subject and other health care units that have blood banks.

DELIMITATION

The present research study will be developed temporarily in the period framed from July 2019 to July 2020, in the blood bank of the Coromoto Hospital of Maracaibo-Venezuela.

FEASIBILITY

This study will be feasible because we have the human resources, equipment and support of the respective authorities of the Coromoto Hospital of Maracaibo, Zulia State, Venezuela, to carry it out. Having the support of the Bioethics department of the institution who granted the permission for the development of this research.

CHAPTER 2: THEORETICAL FRAMEWORK

CONCEPTUAL THEORETICAL FRAMEWORK

RESEARCH BACKGROUND

Montero (Venezuela, 2019) *"Coinfections in blood donors in blood bank of Coromoto Hospital: 2018-2019",* carried out a non-experimental, descriptive, retrospective and cross-sectional research work, in which the histories of donors seropositive for blood-borne diseases such as Chagas, Syphilis, hepatitis B, hepatitis C, as well as those transmitted through HIV and HTLVI were reviewed. Of 11976 donors attended during the study period 341 (2.85%) were positive for STIs, being more frequent in the male sex 316 (92.67%) and these in turn presented coinfections 10 (3.16%) the seropositivity mostly found was for syphilis- Anti core tests 4 (1,27%), followed by syphilis-HIV 2 (0.63%), syphilis-HBs-Ag 1 (0.32%), Chagas - Syphilis 1 (0.32%), Chagas - anti core 1 (0.32%) and Syphilis - HbsAg - anti core 1 (0.32%) representing 3.16% of the total population[11] .

Vizcaya-Rodriguez (Venezuela, 2019) *"Prevalence of transfusion-transmissible infections in the south of Lara state, Venezuela",* conducted a research work whose objective was to determine the prevalence of any transfusion-transmitted infection in blood donors who attended the Dr. Egidio Montesinos Hospital in the city of El Tocuyo during the years 2010-2017. In this study, 6440 sera were analyzed by ELISA test from different biotechnological companies, of which 481 cases have been reactive to different infections which yields a 7.47% prevalence to any transfusion-transmitted infection; A seroprevalence of 0.66% for HBsAg, for anti-HBc (5.34%), for HCV (0.17%), for *Trypanosoma cruzi* infection (0.42%), for *Treponema pallidum* infection (0.61%) and for HIV (0.26%). No reactive case was found for HTLV[12] .

Badaraco (Venezuela, 2017) *"Risk factors of sexually transmitted infections in blood donors of the Hospital Coromoto de Maracaibo year 2016-2017"* which conducted a descriptive, prospective and cross-sectional research work; with the application of questionnaires specifying that most of these infections occur in young men and early adults, through inadequate social and sexual behaviors. A population of 12,816 donors who came to the blood bank of the Coromoto Hospital of Maracaibo during this period of time was studied; of which 540 were positive to any of the serological tests, either HIV, syphilis or HBV, and only 264 participated in the surveys. The results were that 81% of the donors were men aged between 13-30 years; 4.21% of the subjects were positive to one or more of the tests, the most frequent being HBV with 2% of the donors, followed by syphilis in 1.74% and finally HIV infection present in only 0.40%[13]

.

Urrutia Jiménez (Mexico, 2016) *"Seroprevalence and sociodemographic characteristics of importance in blood donors with screening tests reactive to HBV, HCV and HIV, in the Central Blood Bank CMN La Raza"*. Who conducted an observational, retrospective, cross-sectional, descriptive study; in order to know the seroprevalence and sociodemographic characteristics of donors who present reactive screening tests to HBV, HCV and HIV in the Central Blood Bank Centro Medico Nacional La Raza, 500,473 donors of the BCS CMN LA RAZA were analyzed, during the period from January 2011 to December 2015. The highest seroprevalence was observed for HCV with 0.055%, followed by HIV with 0.039% and finally HBV with 0.027%. The most important sociodemographic characteristics in the donors with positive serology for the viral agents studied were age group, schooling and marital status. The hepatotropic viruses presented similar characteristics, such as age over 41 years, married marital status, and secondary schooling. HIV had a different behavior, with a higher frequency in the group under 40 years of age, single marital status and higher education[14] .

Daza Bolaño, N. (Colombia, 2016). *"Prevalence of infections in blood donors at the Universidad Industrial de Santander versus parks in the city of Bucaramanga, 2014"* a cross-sectional study was conducted in which 3758 results of blood donations in blood collection campaigns in the Plaza Cívica, Santander and San Pío parks in the metropolitan area of Bucaramanga were evaluated. Subsequently, they were analyzed in the blood bank of the Hospital Universitario de Santander, to determine the prevalence of infections transmitted by blood transfusion, analyzed in the study; syphilis, Human T-Cell Lymphotropic Virus, HIV, Chagas, Hepatitis B and C. The results obtained were: 187 positive serologies in total, with 78 positive cases of syphilis, 20 of Chagas, 81 of Hepatitis B, 13 of Hepatitis C, 6 of HIV, and 10 of HTLV[15] .

Salas Ponce, P. (Peru, 2015) *"Seroprevalence of markers of transfusion-transmissible infections in the Blood Bank of the Hospital Nacional Arzobispo Loayza in the period January 2011 and December 2014".* The results show that the base population consisted of 34245 donors, 8.97% presented at least one positive screening test. The most prevalent markers were HBcAc (4.6%), syphilis (1.88%) and HTLV (0.89%), followed by HIV (0.17%), Hepatitis B surface antigen (0.36%), Chagas (0.25%), Hepatitis C (0.82%). He concluded that the prevalences found coincide with those reported in other national studies[16] .

Concepción-Zavaleta, M (Peru, 2014) *"Frequency of serological markers of infections transmissible by blood transfusion in voluntary donors in a hospital in Trujillo, Peru 2014".* They designed a cross-sectional study, in which they evaluated 6,000 donors, of which, by self-exclusion and physical examination, 4,000 donors remained, of which 10% were voluntary donors, so 418 voluntary donors were considered as sample size in the study. The results showed a prevalence rate of seropositivity in blood donors of 2.4%. Hepatitis B virus had the highest prevalence with a rate of 1.44%. The second most frequent cause of seropositivity was syphilis, with a prevalence rate of 0.72%. The prevalence rates for HIV, HCV, and HTLV I-II were 0.24 % for each.
The prevalence rate of Chagas disease was 0%. Therefore, it is concluded that the prevalence of diseases transmissible by blood transfusion in the locality does not differ significantly from that found in the rest of the hospitals in the country[17] .

Jeél Moya and Edward Julcamanyan (Peru, 2014) *"Seroprevalence of infectious markers causing hemodonation losses in the Blood Bank Service of the Hospital Nacional Docente Madre Niño San Bartolomé from January 2008 to December 2013"* Objective: To determine the seroprevalence of infectious markers causing hemodonation losses in the Blood Bank Service of the Hospital Nacional Docente Madre-Niño San Bartolomé from January 2008 to December 2013. Material and Methods: Retrospective, cross-sectional, descriptive study. The inclusion criterion was complete hemodonations without complications that met the quality and normative criteria of PRONAHEBAS. Data analysis was performed in three basic processes: coding, tabulation and construction of tables and graphs. The technique used for statistical verification of the results was SPSS version 20.0 statistical analyzer. Results: The findings were: 4.63% for HBcAb, 1.78% for syphilis, 1.21% for HTLV I-II, and 5.31% for other serological markers out of a total of 11399 complete donations. The overall prevalence was 9.36% for all markers, resulting in a loss of 1016 donations; 457.2 liters of blood and 61,893.28 USD lost. The associations between the most frequent infectious markers were: HBcAb with syphilis and HBsAg and the three components that explain the variance were associated by chronicity and epidemics concentrated in populations, by occupational exposure and by subrogating relationship. Conclusion: The prevalence found showed the poor quality of blood donors and the great economic impact of discarded blood derivatives show the limitations in the donation chain. It is therefore advisable to continue with health education campaigns, good practices in transfusion medicine and the selection of blood donors to prevent transfusion-transmissible infections, increase the blood supply without putting the recipient at risk and without new donations, and reduce the economic cost lost per donation[18] .

Flores Pichardo (Mexico, 2014) *"Prevalence of hepatitis B in whole blood donors of the Blood Bank of the Hospital General Regional 25 identified through simultaneous HBsAG and Anti-HBc tests"* This is an observational, comparative, cross-sectional, retrospective study in which a review of the results of viral serology of whole blood donors of the BSHGR25 was performed, having as results that during the study period from January 2005 to December 2012, 47.012 donors were registered in the BSHGR25, of which 71 presented reactivity to HBsAg, calculating a prevalence of 0.15% of donors with reactivity to this marker[19] .

Ortiz Arauz (Ecuador, 2014). *"Seroprevalence of blood-borne infectious diseases in donors attending blood bank of the Enrique C. Sotomayor Maternity Hospital from January 2006 to December 2012"* This research was conducted with the objective of establishing the seroprevalence of infectious markers of blood samples from 68,909 apparently healthy donors who attended the Enrique C. Sotomayor Maternity Blood Bank of Guayaquil from January 2006 to December 2012. A statistical analysis of the software of the Blood Bank of the Junta de Beneficencia de Guayaquil was performed, all donors were included of which 2226 were positive for any pathogen, the samples were analyzed by the third and fourth generation ELISA method to identify surface antigen (HBsAg), Hepatitis C virus (HCV) antibodies, human immunodeficiency virus (HIV) antibodies, cytomegalovirus (CMV) antibodies, *Trypanosoma cruzi* antibodies *and* syphilis treponemal antibodies (VDRL). Results: The following prevalence was determined: VDRL (1.23%), HCV (0.32%), HBV (0.58%), CMV (0.26%), HIV (0.37%) and Chagas disease (0.46%). In addition, the population classified as being at high risk of transmitting infections was from the province of Guayas and was male[20].

THEORETICAL BASIS

TRANSFUSION-TRANSMITTED INFECTIOUS DISEASES

The risk of blood transfusion of bacterial infectious diseases is more frequent in developed countries, but for developing countries, the incidence is the same for any infectious agent, whether viral, bacterial or parasitic; this is due to the geographical diversity, types of habitat and population groups, where studies have been carried out and the percentage of infections by transfusion of blood and its derivatives is not very encouraging[16].

The first cases of transfusion of viral infections in the world were reported in 1943 and laboratory studies for blood screening began in 1969, with the identification of hepatitis B virus (HBV) surface antigen, but at present, transfusion of blood components still cannot be performed without some residual risk[21].

Although it has not been possible to achieve total control to prevent the transmission of transfusion-transfused infections, the World Health Organization (WHO) has been vigilant in ensuring that all blood material and blood products from voluntary donors are screened for infectious markers and that priority is given to the processing to determine: Hepatitis B virus surface antigen (AgHBs) and Core antigen (anti-HBc), antibodies to HIV type I and/or II (anti-HIV1 and anti-HIV 2), antibodies to hepatitis C virus (anti-HCV) and syphilis serology[21] .

Likewise, it is essential to take into account the lack of programs and education of the population by the local health organizations in charge of this type of transfusion-transmitted diseases, which are generally also sexually transmitted, which is what causes the number of transfusion-transmitted infections to rise every day without any real commitment on the part of these organizations and the individuals of the affected community. Therefore, with a better control of transfusion-transmissible diseases, it is possible to count on this therapeutic method that helps to save lives, since it is a mechanism used in emergency situations in hospital institutions around the world[21] .

Another important aspect is that transfusion-transmissible infections are very varied and if a review is made, it is clear that in studies carried out and published, four new viruses have been reported since 1995, which are also transmissible by blood transfusion, such as Hepatitis G virus (HHV), Transfusion Transmissible Virus (TTV), Human Herpes Virus Type 8 (HHV-8) and SEN-V2[22] .

Among the group of biological agents that meet the criteria to be grouped as microorganisms causing infections by transfusion transmission we have Viruses: Hepatitis B virus (HBV), hepatitis C virus (HCV), hepatitis A virus (HAV), hepatitis D virus (HDV), hepatitis E virus (HEV), human immunodeficiency virus (HIV 1 and 2), HTLV I/II, cytomegalovirus, Epstein-Barr virus (EBV), parvovirus B 19, SARS, TTV, West Nile virus; Parasites: *Plasmodium, Trypanosoma cruzi, Babesia microfti, Leishmania, Toxoplasma gondii;* Bacteria: *Staphylococcus aureus, B. diphtheroides,* micrococci, *Pseudomonas aeruginosa,* acromobacteria, coliforms, *Salmonella, Yersinia enterocolitica, Serratia marsenses, Treponema pallidum, Brucella, Borrelia burgdorferi;* Others: Prions[23] .

In the present study, when mentioning transfusion-transmitted diseases, reference is made to mandatory screening diseases caused by biological agents such as HIV, hepatitis B virus, hepatitis C virus, HTLV-1, the spirochete *Treponema pallidum* and the *Trypanozoma cruzi* parasite, which are reviewed below:

HUMAN IMMUNODEFICIENCY VIRUS (HIV)

It is a Lentivirus that has a predilection for infecting CD4 lymphocytes, presents an aggressive replication and becomes chronic. Due to its lymphotropism, it triggers a marked immunosuppression in the host, not so much by the destruction of CD4 lymphocytes, but by the interference it causes in the immune system, causing infections by opportunistic germs, neurological disorders and cancer, which is known as immunodeficiency syndrome (AIDS)[24] .

Pathophysiology develops from virus entry into the cell and interaction with CD4 and chemokine receptors CCR5 or CXCR4; initially interacts with gp120 and CD4 receptor induces

Conformational changes and exposes V3 domain that form the gp120 binding domain and chemokine receptors; this causes new changes in the structure of gp41 that exposes the N-terminal region and allows it to anchor to the plasma membrane. Once the viral and cell membranes are fused, internalization of the nucleocapsid and release of the viral genome occurs[24] .

The process of DNA synthesis from viral RNA or retrotranscription is carried out by the reverse transcriptase enzyme complex, but, in an unactivated lymphocyte, retrotranscription occurs incompletely and is degraded within 3 to 15 days by cellular nucleases. It is necessary to activate the infected cell to complete the synthesis; once the proviral DNA is completed, the pre-integration complex is formed and transported to the nucleus of the host cell, where it is integrated into the genome and forms the HIV provirus. The non-integrated DNA, which is approximately 90% of the viral

DNA, constitutes the reservoir in circulating lymphocytes, awaiting activation to complete the cycle[24] .

The main cellular factor involved in the transition from viral latency to reactivation is NF-κB, a family of proteins that regulate the expression of multiple cellular genes involved in immune recognition and activation processes. This factor does not exist in active form in CD4 lymphocytes in the resting state and is induced in the course of immune activation processes[24] .

HEPATITIS B VIRUS

Hepatitis B virus is a hepatotropic DNA virus, belonging to the *Hepadnaviridae* family. It has the capacity to infect humans, being man the only reservoir with the capacity to infect others; it has a sphere shape with a lipoprotein shell formed by several proteins, among which the main one is the surface antigen S (HBsAg). This shell surrounds the capsid formed by the *core* antigen (HBcAg) and a series of soluble excreted HBcAg-like proteins formed by the e antigen (HBeAg). The capsid encloses the virus genome, the DNA polymerase[25] .

HBV enters the hepatocyte by binding of surface proteins to receptors on the cell itself, subsequently releasing the capsid into the cytoplasm. In the cytoplasm the virus is decapsidated and its DNA is transported to the nucleus. Initially it is converted into double-stranded circular DNA closed by covalent bonds (DNAccc) due to the action of polymerases of the virus and the host[25] .

Hepatitis B virus infection is one of the most frequent infectious diseases in the world and with the widest geographical distribution. HBV is responsible for a high rate of morbidity and mortality worldwide, whether due to acute (fulminant hepatitis) or chronic (cirrhosis or hepatocarcinoma) infection, it presents specific serological patterns depending on the stage of infection. The serological markers routinely used are determined by enzyme-linked immunosorbent assay (ELISA) and include: HBsAg, anti-HBs, anti-HBc (total and IgM), HBeAg and anti-HBe[25] .

HEPATITIS C VIRUS

Hepatitis C virus is an RNA virus, of the *Flaviviradae* family, genus *Hepacivirus,* whose replication is exclusive in hepatocytes and as it is not a cytopathic virus, it acquires the particularity of being a virus that causes chronic persistent disease. The HCV virion has an RNA genome, surrounded by an icosahedral capsid (Core) and an envelope containing 2 glycoproteins, E1 and E2. The viral particles are approximately 50 nm in diameter and the Core around 30 nm; the RNA functions as a messenger and its translation leads to a polyprotein precursor from which the different functional proteins, structural and non-structural, are produced by the action of cellular proteases and viral coding[26] .

A very important characteristic of HCV is the genetic variability or high degree of heterogeneity in the genomic sequences and, therefore, of the encoded proteins. This particularity of the virus makes it persistent in the design of vaccines and the design and interpretation of diagnostic methods. For the detection of antibodies, enzyme immunoassay (EIA) techniques are normally used, as they are inexpensive, convenient to perform and, moreover, are adapted to today's automated systems; as for molecular methods, quantitative tests for measuring viral load and genotyping are used to evaluate HCV disease and to establish a prognosis on the efficacy of treatment and to monitor the response to treatment[26] .

HUMAN LYMPHOTROPIC VIRUS TYPE 1 (HTLV-1)

The human lymphotropic virus type 1 (HTLV-1) belongs to the *Retroviridae* family *and* to the *Oncovirinae* subfamily, which is characterized by the involvement of CD4 lymphocytes, and is therefore related to complications such as lymphoma and T-cell leukemia in adults. Particularly, the concentration of the virus in plasma is quite low, so the contagion takes place when there is contact with infected lymphocytes, which can be through prolonged breastfeeding, sexual intercourse and blood transfusions[8] .

It is well known that its main complication is neoplastic diseases; however, by interfering with the reproduction of T lymphocytes, it can cause various inflammatory pathologies as a result of this dysfunction (such as tropical spastic paraparesis, uveitis, thyroiditis and alveolitis), as well as infectious complications (strongyloidiasis, scabies, tuberculosis, among others)[8] .

Treponema pallidum (SIFILIS)

Treponema pallidum subspecies *pallidum.* It is a very fine spirochete, which cannot be observed by Gram staining; *T. pallidum* does not grow in bacteriological culture media, is sensitive to desiccation and is rapidly inactivated by disinfectant agents. This microorganism has the peculiarity that it is not cytopathic, possesses non-toxic lipopolysaccharides (LPS) and does not possess exotoxins, nor does it release products with enzymatic activity[27] .

Its evasion mechanism is represented by its ability to form an insoluble layer and cover itself with host proteins in order to evade the immune system. It adheres to the fibronectin of the monocytes by means of an adhesin that it possesses and this union causes the activation of adhesion molecules of the monocytes and the initiation of a process that leads to obliterative endoarteritis of small vessels. The binding of these receptors produces a response of the host immune system, where it does not know its own fibronectin, a humoral response is generated, antibodies that attack host tissues and thus *Treponema pallidum* has the ability to cross tissues, including placenta[27] .

Trypanosoma cruzi (CHAGAS DISEASE)

Chagas disease (also known as American trypanosomiasis) can be described as a parasitemia caused by the protozoan *Trypanosoma cruzi.* The main route of transmission is through triatomines such as *Rhodnius prolixus, Triatoma maculata and Panstrongylus geniculatus,* mainly in Venezuela[28] .

This form of transmission occurs by contact of triatomine fecal matter containing parasites with the skin orifice produced by the insect's bite to suck blood, or by deposition of feces on the host's mucous membranes. Oral transmission is also possible through the ingestion of contaminated food. There are also other routes such as blood transfusion, congenital transmission, organ transplantation and transmission related to laboratory or occupational accidents in health care workers[28] .

BASIC TERMS

INFECTION: A phenomenon that occurs in the presence of a pathogenic agent, characterized by an inflammatory response to the presence of microorganisms, or the invasion of normally sterile host tissues by these[29] .

TRANSFUSION-BORNE INFECTIONS: Transfusion-transmissible infections to be grouped in this category and represent a danger to public health must meet certain biological characteristics, among others, it must be present in the blood and transmitted parenterally in an effective way, it must belong to the group of endemic diseases in the donor population, it must be a stable biological agent in the conditions of conservation of blood components and the biological agent must cause a defined disease[30]
.

VOLUNTARY DONOR: A voluntary donor is a person with a social and empathic sense, who understands the need for blood donations, who donates blood, plasma or blood derivative by decision and will, without receiving any payment or reward. Their motivation is to help others and they do not obtain any personal benefit[17] .

THEORETICAL AND OPERATIONAL FRAMEWORK

HYPOTHESIS

Blood-borne infectious diseases are frequent in blood donors of the Coromoto Hospital of Maracaibo, in the period July 2019 to July 2020.

VARIABLE SYSTEM

Dependent Variables: Serology for HIV, HBsAg, anti-HBc, HCV, HTLV-1, syphilis and Chagas disease.
Independent variables: age, sex, origin.

TRANSFUSION-TRANSMITTED DISEASES

Conceptual Definition: According to the World Health

Organization (WHO) and the Pan American Health Organization (PAHO) are considered transfusion-transmitted diseases, infectious processes transmitted through blood and blood products being of greater relevance for being a public health problem, Human immunodeficiency virus (HIV), Hepatitis B virus (HBV), Hepatitis C virus (HCV), human lymphotropic virus type 1 (HTLV-1), syphilis *(Treponema pallidum) and* Chagas disease *(Trypanosoma cruzi)*.

Operational Definition: Samples from apparently healthy volunteer donors Seropositive for Human Immunodeficiency Virus (HIV), Hepatitis B Virus (HBV), Hepatitis V virus (HCV), human lymphotropic virus type 1 (HTLV-1), *Treponema pallidum* and *Trypanosoma cruzi.*

HUMAN IMMUNODEFICIENCY VIRUS (HIV)

Conceptual Definition: Human immunodeficiency virus (HIV) is a lentivirus of the *Retroviridae family, which* causes Acquired Immunodeficiency Syndrome (AIDS). The infection is characterized by a progressive depression of the immune system due to the virus attacking the cells of the host organism, mainly CD4+ T lymphocytes. Two strains are known in the world, HIV1 and HIV-2. The virus has been isolated from most human body fluids[24] .

Operational Definition: The Human Immunodeficiency Virus (HIV) consists of two recognized strains (HIV-1 and HIV-2). The diagnosis will be made at the moment of a positive reaction to the fourth generation ELISA test (HIV) in two opportunities, according to the brand available at the Blood Bank of the Hospital Coromoto de Maracaibo (for example: Litmus®, Stadia®, Bioline®, Murex®).

HEPATITIS B VIRUS (HBV)

Conceptual Definition: Hepatitis B is a life-threatening liver infection caused by the hepatitis B virus (HBV). It can cause chronic liver disease and carries a high risk of death from cirrhosis and liver cancer. The virus is transmitted by contact with the blood or other body fluids of an infected person[25] .

Operational Definition: Hepatitis B virus (HBV) infection is characterized by high serum HBV DNA levels; the diagnosis of acute hepatitis B is based on the detection of HBsAg and anti-HBc, according to the brand available at the Blood Bank of the Hospital Coromoto de Maracaibo (e.g. Litmus®, Stadia®, Bioline®, Murex®).

HEPATITIS C VIRUS (HCV)

Conceptual Definition: Hepatitis C virus (HCV) has an RNA genome, of the *Flaviviridae family,* surrounded by an icosahedral capsid (Core) and an envelope containing 2 glycoproteins, E1 and E2. Due to its ability to persist even in the presence of a good humoral and cellular immune response of the host, a consequence of the high mutation rate that facilitates escape mechanisms as well as the high production and clearance of HCV virions, it is considered a severe infection[26] .

Operational Definition: By fourth generation ELISA method, according to the brand available at the Blood Bank of the Hospital Coromoto de Maracaibo (for example: Litmus®, Stadia®, Bioline®, Murex®).

HTLV-1

Conceptual Definition: HTLV-1 belongs to the *Retroviridae* family *and* to the *Oncovirinae* subfamily*, and* is characterized by the involvement of CD4 lymphocytes, which is why it is related to neoplastic complications, as well as inflammatory syndromes and infectious complications in a minority of patients who may present manifestations[8] .

Operational definition: antibodies against the virus are detected through fourth generation ELISA tests, according to the brand available at the Blood Bank of the Hospital Coromoto de Maracaibo (for example: Litmus®, Stadia®, Bioline®, Murex®).

SYPHILIS

Conceptual Definition: Syphilis is an infectious disease with systemic involvement caused by the microorganism *Treponema pallidum* subspecies *pallidum,* belonging to the Order *Spirochaetales,* family *Spirochaetaceae.* The infection caused is syphilis, which can be acquired by sexual contact, congenitally through the placenta, by transfusion of contaminated human blood and by direct accidental inoculation[27] .

Operational definition: antibodies against the spirochete are detected by fourth generation ELISA, according to the brand available at the Blood Bank of the Hospital Coromoto de Maracaibo (for example: Litmus®, Stadia®, Bioline®, Murex®).

CHAGAS DISEASE

Conceptual Definition: Trypanosomiasis is caused by the protozoan *Trypanosoma cruzi.* This pathology is characterized by an acute clinical presentation that can be symptomatic, oligosymptomatic or asymptomatic. In chronic cases, cardiological, digestive and neurological manifestations may be evident[28] .

Operational definition: the method for parasite detection is with fourth generation ELISA, according to the brand available at the Blood Bank of the Hospital Coromoto de Maracaibo (for example: Litmus®, Stadia®, Bioline®, Murex®).

SYSTEMATIZATION OF VARIABLES

General Objective: To determine the seroprevalence of blood-borne infectious diseases in blood bank donors of the Coromoto Hospital of Maracaibo-Venezuela, from July 2019 to July 2020.				
Objectives	Variables	Dimensions	Indicators	Categories

| To determine the frequency of each of the blood-borne diseases in donors of the blood bank of the Coromoto Hospital of Maracaibo-Venezuela, in the period 20192020. | Transfusion transmitted diseases

VHB

HCV

HIV

HTLV-1

SYPHILIS

CHAGAS | Indicators

Immunological and Serological | ELISA | Qualitative

POSITIVE

NEGATIVE |
| To determine the distribution of donors with positive serology for sexually transmitted infections according to sex. | Sex | Survey | Male

Female | Qualitative |

| To determine the distribution of donors with positive serology for sexually transmitted infections according to age. | Age in years | Survey | Age groups | Qualitative |
| To determine the distribution of donors with positive serology for sexually transmitted infections according to origin. | Origin by municipality or state | Survey | Municipality in the state of Zulia from which it originates | Qualitative |

Determine if there is a relationship between the presence of blood-borne infectious diseases in	Relationship between variables	Relationship between variables	Chi-square	Qualitative $p<0,05$
donors of		qualitative	Correlation of	Direct

blood bank of the Coromoto Hospital of Maracaibo-Venezuela, in the period July 2019 to July 2020 and the sociodemographic variables of the same.		Correlation 29	Spearman	Indirect

CHAPTER 3: METHODOLOGICAL FRAMEWORK

TYPE OF RESEARCH

The present study is a retrospective, cross-sectional, non-experimental, descriptive, retrospective study.

RESEARCH DESIGN

The research design is non-experimental and cross-sectional.

POPULATION AND SAMPLE

The total population is constituted by voluntary donor users attending the Blood Bank of the Coromoto Hospital of Maracaibo in the period July 2019-July 2020. Who meet the inclusion and exclusion criteria of the study.

DATA COLLECTION

INCLUSION AND EXCLUSION CRITERIA:

INCLUSION CRITERIA

- Of both genders without distinction of ethnic group.
- Individuals weighing more than 55 kg.
- Age between 18 and 60 years old.
- No associated pathologies: cardiovascular, metabolic, autoimmune.
- To sign the informed consent form.

EXCLUSION CRITERIA

- Donors under 18 years of age and over 60 years of age.
- Individuals weighing less than 55 kg
- With clinical history of any sexually transmitted disease.
- Individuals with tattoos and/or piercings.
- Women, not pregnant, breastfeeding or menstruating
- That they express their desire not to continue in the study.

INSTRUMENTS

In this research, a data collection form was elaborated that included: clinical history: age, gender, place of residence, laboratory tests.

PROCEDURE AND METHODS

SAMPLE COLLECTION

Blood samples were obtained by venous puncture, collected in tubes without anticoagulants and centrifuged at 3000 r.p.m. for 10 minutes to obtain serum and subsequent analysis.

DATA ANALYSIS

The results obtained were entered into an Excel spreadsheet for subsequent statistical analysis. The average and standard deviation of the quantitative and qualitative values were calculated. The final results are expressed in graphs, by number, percentage and absolute values. Qualitative variables were analyzed using Pearson's chi-square test. The confidence index was 95% and a probability value of less than 0.05 ($p<0.05$) was considered significant. For this purpose, the statistical program SPSS for Windows, version 21.0, 2014, was used. Chicago, Illinois, USA.

ETHICAL CONSIDERATIONS

This research complies with the four principles of bioethics, which were established by Beauchamp and Childress in 1979 with the purpose of regulating respect for human beings and all their rights.

In this order of ideas, the first principle, respect for autonomy, will be fulfilled since the privacy of the individuals who will be part of this study will be respected, as the data will not be disclosed.

The data collected were also used with their personal data and they were informed of their use by means of an informed consent form.

The next of the principles, nonmaleficence, will be executed by not intentionally inflicting death, pain, injury or suffering on the donors who will be part of the study.

Following with justice, since all data collected in this research will be done without distinction of gender, ethnicity, culture, ideology or social class, providing all donors with the same conditions.

And finally, there is the charitable basis, since the results of this research will be useful for both public health providers and epidemiological surveillance authorities, who together will be able to provide care to the communities most affected by these diseases.

The study will be reviewed and approval will be sought from the Bioethics Committee of the Military Academy of Medicine (AMMED) and the Coromoto Hospital of Maracaibo. For the subsequent storage of the sample data, the voluntary collaboration of the population and authorities will be requested, emphasizing the confidentiality of the study.

CHAPTER 4: ADMINISTRATIVE FRAMEWORK

HUMAN RESOURCES

Name	Profession	Institution	Cargo	Responsibility
ALF.AUX/VI Angélica Mujica	Medical Student	Academy Military of Medicine	Thesis writer	Author
GM/VI Genesis Bolivar	Medical Student	Academy Military of Medicine	Thesis writer	Author
Dr. Rafael Villalobos	D. in Medical Sciences	Military Academy of Medicine Coromoto Hospital	Research Professor	Academic tutor and statistical analysis
Dr. Ricardo Attention	D. in Biological Sciences	Military Academy of Medicine Coromoto Hospital	Researcher	Methodological Tutor

MATERIAL RESOURCE
- Injectors
- Cotton
- Alcohol
- Fourth generation ELISA tests, according to availability

INSTITUTIONAL RESOURCES
- Maracaibo Coromoto Hospital Blood Bank
- Military Academy of Medicine

SCHEDULE OF ACTIVITIES

N°	ACTIVITIES	DATE
1.	Project Reception (AMMED Research Unit)	28/06/20-10/07/20
2.	Project review (AMMED Academic Committee)	11/07/20-15/09/20
3.	Delivery of the Approval of the projects to the thesis students (AMMED Academic Committee).	15/09/20-20/09/20
4.	Appointment of jurors (AMMED Research Unit)	20/09/20-25/09/20
5.	Submission of projects to the Bioethics Committee of the different Hospitals (AMMED Research Unit).	25/09/20-30/09/20
6.	Progress Report (Problem Statement, Theoretical Framework, Legal Framework, Methodological Framework)	15/11/20-30/11/20
7.	Review of progress (AMMED Research Unit)	01/12/20-10/12/20
8.	Delivery of progress (Instrument, Results, Discussion and Conclusions)	20/01/21-30/01/21
9.	Review of progress (AMMED Research Unit)	31/01/21-10/02/21
10.	Delivery of the final manuscript by the Ensigns to the Research Unit.	15/03/21-01/04/21
11.	Submission of manuscripts to jurors (AMMED Research Unit)	01/04/21-15/04/21
12.	Submission of the jury's considerations	01/05/21-05/05/21
13.	Delivery of corrections to the research unit	20/05/21-25/05/21
14.	Presentation of the special degree work	01/06/21-11/06/21

CHAPTER 5: ANALYSIS OF THE RESULTS

A total of 3846 voluntary donors were studied during the period 2019-2020, of which a total of 133 positive serologies were estimated for any of the screening tests performed at the Coromoto Hospital Blood Bank, which represented 3.45% of the donor population in this period, as shown in Graph N°1.

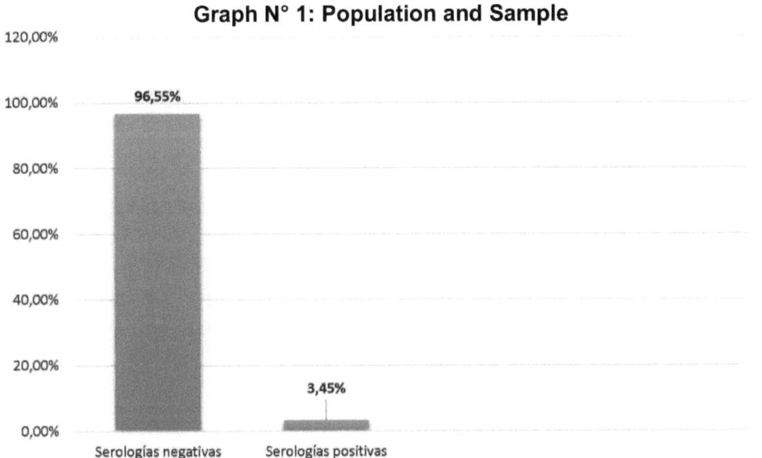

Graph N° 1: Population and Sample

Source: Blood Bank of the Coromoto Hospital of Maracaibo.

Following this order of ideas, 5 cases of donors were documented who were positive for more than one serology, which corresponds to 0.13%. As described in graph n°2.

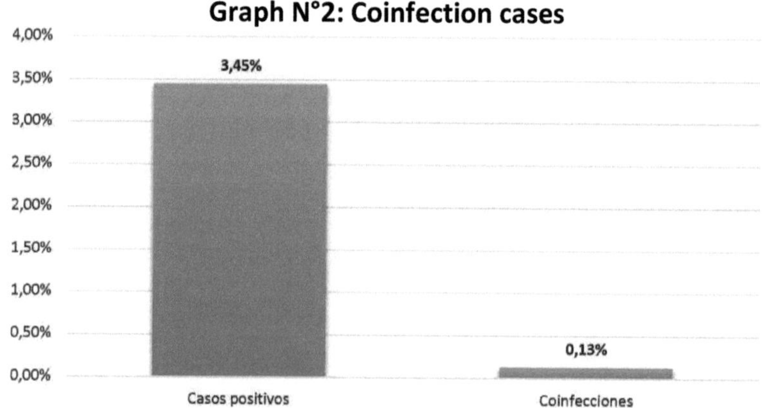

Source: Blood Bank of the Coromoto Hospital of Maracaibo.

Likewise, of the total number of subjects studied, 128 were positive to one or more serologies, with a total of 121 male cases, which corresponds to 94.5%, as opposed to the remaining 7 female cases (5.5%), as shown in graph N°3.

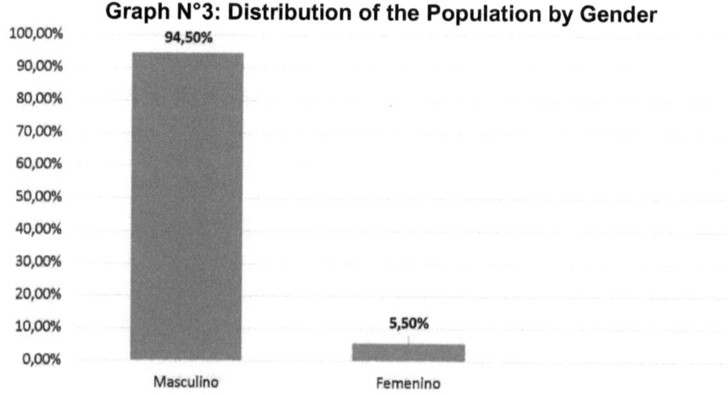

Source: Blood Bank of the Coromoto Hospital of Maracaibo.

Graph 4 shows the distribution according to each age group, with the highest percentage of positive cases (32%) in individuals aged 36 to 45 years, corresponding to 41 cases; followed by the groups aged 26 to 35 years and 46 to 60 years, with a total of 35 cases each (27.3%); and 13.3% in the group aged 18 to 25 years, with 17 cases in the latter group.

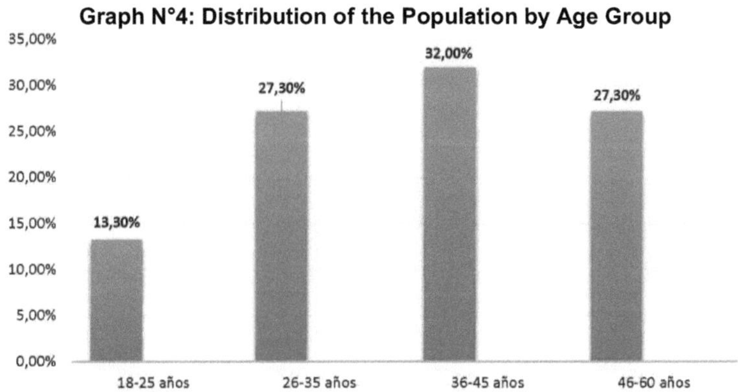

Graph N°4: Distribution of the Population by Age Group

Source: Blood Bank of the Coromoto Hospital of Maracaibo.

With respect to the total number of positive cases for any of the serologies studied according to their origin, the most relevant municipality was Maracaibo with 79 cases, representing 61.7% of the total sample; followed by Cabimas with 11 cases, which translates to 8.6%; In third place was the municipality of San Francisco with a total of 8 cases, representing 6.3%; followed by Santa Rita, Los Puertos and Mara with 5 cases, equivalent to 3.9% each; then Simón Bolívar, La Cañada and those from other states of the country, had 3 cases, representing 2.3%. The rest of the municipalities mentioned above had 1 case, equivalent to 0.8% of the sample under study, as shown in Graph 5.

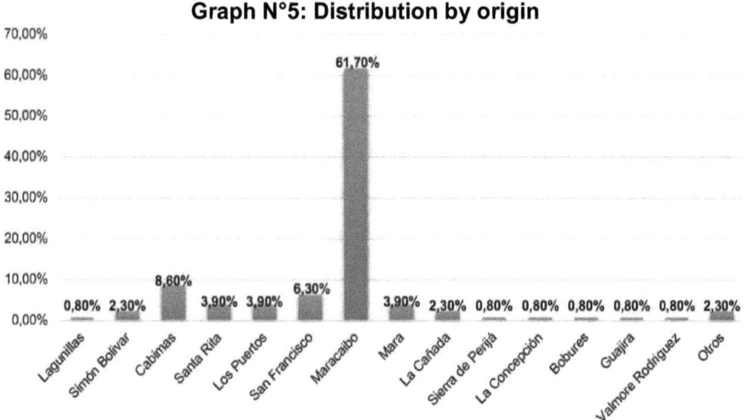

Source: Blood bank of the Coromoto Hospital of Maracaibo.

On the other hand, of the total number of samples studied, 133 positive serologies were obtained (3.45%), represented in graph n°6, of which 63 serologies corresponded to Syphilis (1.63%), obtaining the highest number of cases; 53 samples for anti-HBc (1.37%); 6 for HIV (0.15%); 4 cases with HbsAg (0.10%); 3 serologies for both Chagas and HCV (0.07%); and finally HTLV-1 with 1 case (0.02%).

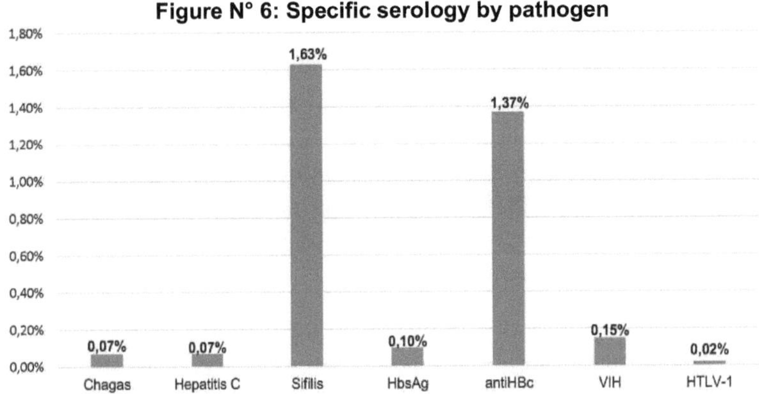

Source: Blood bank of the Coromoto Hospital of Maracaibo.

CHAPTER 6 : DISCUSSION, CONCLUSIONS AND RECOMMENDATIONS

It is well known that blood transfusions are a widely used means in different medical services to save or improve the quality of life of the patient who receives them. Blood banks are the entities in charge of receiving and ensuring the correct administration of blood from voluntary donors who come to them. The blood bank of the Coromoto Hospital, due to the great demand by the specialties, both medical and surgical, that are performed in this center, handles high amounts of donors; however, the influx was considerably decreased with respect to previous years, demonstrated in previous studies conducted in this institution who report a total of 12816 donors in the period from 2016-2017[13] , and, 11976 donors between 2018-2019[11] , unlike the 3846 reflected in this study.

Likewise, the difference between the figures for each gender of donors who tested positive for serology is noteworthy, where the male gender obtained 94.5% of the cases, marking a significant gap to the 5.5% represented by the female gender, which may be explained by the lower number of female donors who meet the inclusion criteria established by the WHO.

On the other hand, when studying the origin of the subjects who tested positive for any of the serologies, it was found that the majority (60.1%) came from the municipality of Maracaibo, which could be explained by the geographical location of the Coromoto Hospital. In second place was Cabimas (8.6%), due to the fact that, being an oil-producing municipality and a hospital attached to the Health Service of PDVSA (Petróleos De Venezuela Sociedad Anónima), most of the patients who work for this institution are transferred to this health center.

In terms of age, the average is considered to be 38.7 ± 10.23 years; similarly, it was observed that the most affected were in the age group of 36 to 45 years, with 32%; unlike a similar study conducted in this hospital center where the most affected donors were between 18 and 40 years, with 70%[13] .

Taking into account the importance of screening tests that include serologies for pathogens that cause blood-borne infections, which, despite being preventable diseases, continue to have a significant prevalence, as described in this work, where 3.45% of the serologies performed in the blood bank of the Coromoto Hospital in the period 2019-2020, were positive for one or more of the tests; unlike previous studies, where 2.85% were obtained[11] .

It is necessary to highlight the finding of 5 subjects (0.13%), who were positive for two serological tests, in contrast to a work performed in this institution during the period 2018-2019[11] , where 10 cases (0.08%) were documented.

Regarding the specific serologies for each pathogen studied, it was recorded that the highest incidence corresponded to syphilis (1.63%); which suggests a relationship with the most prevalent age group, being the population with the greatest accessibility to blood banks, and who are sexually active; The results are similar to those obtained in previous years in this center, where despite occupying second place in incidence, 1.74% was obtained[13] , as well as in another study carried out in the state of Lara, where it also occupied second place, but with a lower percentage (0.61%)[12] .

With respect to the markers used to determine the hepatitis B virus, we obtained a higher prevalence of anti-HBc (1.37%) compared to HbsAg (0.10%), which correlates with the prevalences described in other similar studies carried out in Venezuela, where HBsAg represented 0.66% of the cases, as opposed to anti-HBc with 5.34%[12] .

Within this framework, similar results were obtained for HCV and Chagas with 0.07% of the cases studied for each one; unlike other works carried out in Peru, in 2015[16] , where the prevalence for Chagas was 0.25% and HCV 0.82%, and in 2014[17] , which reported 0.24% for HCV, and 0% for Chagas. In this context, it is necessary to alert public health entities regarding the monitoring of these cases and prevention, emphasizing the correct sanitary control of at-risk areas.

In spite of being an infrequent virus, one case of HTLV-1 (0.02%) was diagnosed, however, there are no studies where the prevalence of this pathogen at the national level can be appreciated; in contrast to studies carried out in Colombia where 10 cases (0.26%) were obtained[15] .

In view of the above, we recommend the implementation of health promotion programs to encourage the prevention of this type of pathogenic entities, and to strengthen sex education programs, since most of these diseases can be transmitted by this route. Also, to emphasize the performance of screening tests to all individuals who come to the blood bank of the Coromoto de Maracaibo hospital to ensure that the process is carried out correctly.

BIBLIOGRAPHIC REFERENCES

1- Reyesa C, Alcántar G. Evolution of blood transfusion. Journal of the Faculty of Medicine UNAM. 2012; *55*(1): 35-42.

2- Salazar M. Guidelines for the transfusion of blood and its components. Pan American Journal of Public Health. 2003; 13: 183-190.

3- Montiel M, Arias J, Chávez M, Herrera O, Atencio M, Coronel K. Syphilis seroprevalence in donors of the blood bank of the University Hospital of Maracaibo. Period 2012-2014. Kasmera. 2016; 44(2): 88-97.

4- Blejer J, Carreras V, Salamone H. Risk of transfusion-transmitted infections. Medicina (B. Aires). 2002; 62(3): 259-78.

5- Alcivar E. Demonstrating the importance of screening for hepatitis core and hepatitis B by chemiluminescence in blood donors (Doctoral dissertation, Universidad de Guayaquil. Faculty of Medical Sciences. Medical Technology Career). 2014.

6- Echavarría E. Study of antibodies against hepatitis C virus in blood donors and high-risk groups. Acta Med Colomb. 1992; 17: 11-15.

7- Gómez M, Pérez N. History and theories of the emergence of the human immunodeficiency virus. Cuban journal of military medicine. 2009; 38(3-4)

8- Gotuzzo E, Gonzalez E, Verdonck K, Mayer E, Ita F, Clark D. Twenty
Years of research on HTLV-1 and its medical complications in Peru: General perspectives. Peruvian Medical Act. 2010; 27(3): 196-203. Retrieved from
http://www.scielo.org.pe/scielo.php?script=sci_arttext&pid= S1728- 59172010000300008&lng=es&tlng=pt.

9- García P, Grassi B, Fich F, Salvo A, Araya L, Abarzúa F. Diagnosis of *Treponema pallidum* infection in patients with early syphilis and neurosyphilis by polymerase chain reaction. Revista chilena de infectología. 2011; 28(4): 310-

315.

10-   Feliciangeli M. Control of Chagas disease in Venezuela. Past achievements and present challenges. Interciencia. 2009; 34(6): 393-399.

11-   Montero, D. Coinfections in blood donors at Coromoto Hospital blood bank: 2018-2019. Maracaibo: Hospital Coromoto, Blood Bank, Maracaibo- Venezuela, Faculty of Medicine, University of Zulia, Regional Laboratory of Virological Reference; 2019.

12-   Vizcaya T. Prevalence of infections transmissible by transfusion in southern Lara state, Venezuela. Kasmera. 2019; 47(1): 50-58. Retrieved from: https://produccioncientificaluz.org/index.php/kasmera/articl e/view/246 77

13-   Badaraco V. Risk factors for sexually transmitted infections in blood donors of the Coromoto Hospital of Maracaibo year 2016-2017". Maracaibo: Hospital Coromoto, Blood Bank, UBV-HC Medical Specializations Program; 2017.

14-   Urrutia I. Seroprevalence and sociodemographic characteristics of importance in blood donors with reactive screening tests for HBV, HCV and HIV at the CMN La Raza Central Blood Bank (Specialization thesis). National Autonomous University of Mexico, Mexico. 2016. Retrieved from https://repositorio.unam.mx/contenidos/211305

15-   Daza N, Sánchez M, Vanegas T, Ortega I. Prevalence of infections in blood donors at the Universidad Industrial de Santander versus parks in the city of Bucaramanga, 2014. Medicas UIS. 2016; 29(3): 55-60.

16-   Salas, P. Seroprevalencia de infecciones transmisibles por transfusión sanguínea Hospital Nacional Arzobispo Loayza 20112014 (Doctoral dissertation, Thesis to obtain the degree of specialist in Clinical Pathology. Universidad San Martin de Porres). 2015.

17-   Concepción M, Concepción L, Marchena M, Estrada L. Frequency of serological markers of infections transmissible by blood transfusion in voluntary donors in a hospital in Trujillo, Peru. Journal of the Medical Corps of the Almanzor Aguinaga Asenjo Hospital. 2014.

18- Moya J, Julcamanyan E. Seroprevalence of infectious markers causing hemodonation losses in the Blood Bank Service of the Hospital Nacional Docente Madre Niño San Bartolomé from January 2008 to December 2013. Horizonte Médico (Lima). 2014; 14(4): 6-14.

19- Flores M. Prevalence of hepatitis B in blood donors. Total Blood Bank of the Regional General Hospital: 25 identified through simultaneous hbsag and anti-hbc tests (Licentiate Thesis). National Autonomous University of Mexico, Mexico. 2014. Retrieved from. https://repositorio.unam.mx/contenidos/130459

20- Ortiz Á. Seroprevalence of blood-borne infectious diseases in donors attending the Enrique C. Sotomayor maternity hospital blood bank from January 2006 to December 2012. 2014.

21- Medina J. Transfusion-transmitted infectious diseases. International and Mexican overview. Gac. Med. Mexico. 2014; *150:* 78-83.

22- Rivero R. Transmission of viral infections by blood transfusion. Cuban Journal of Hematology, Immunology and Hemotherapy. 2006; 22(2)

23- Sánchez P, Sánchez M, Hernández S, Fariñas A. Active surveillance of infectious diseases in blood donors. Cuban Journal of Hematology, Immunology and Hemotherapy. 2013; 29(1): 82-89.

24- Montoya C, Moreno M, Rugeles M. Reactions and alterations of the immune system during HIV-1 infection. Infection. 2006; 10(4): 250-265.

25- Romero G. Hepatitis B. Gen. 2008; *62*(1): 68-73. Retrieved October 25, 2020, from http://ve.scielo.org/scielo.php?script=sci_arttext&pid=S001 6- 35032008000100019&lng=en&tlng=en.

26- Dueñas S, Acosta N, Morales J, García W. Molecular

biology of hepatitis C virus. Mexican Internal Medicine. 2018; 34(3): 435-442. https://doi.org/10.24245/mim.v34i3.1903

27-   Odero M. Study of the clinical-microbiological characteristics of patients with syphilis in the HUVV (Malaga). 2017.

28-   Mitelman J, Descalzo A, Giménez L, Pesce R, Romero H, Auger S. Chagas-Mazza disease consensus. Rev Argent Cardiol. 2011; 79(6): 544-64.

29-   Fariñas A, Dáger A. Sepsis and disorders. related. MEDISAN. 2012; 16(6): 932-948. Retrieved October 25, 2020, from. http://scielo.sld.cu/scielo.php?script=sci_arttext&pid=S102 9- 30192012000600014&lng=es&tlng=es.

30-   Frenes P, Bouza M, Malpica S. Infectious diseases and blood transfusion. 2012

ANNEXES

N°.	Cédula	Age	Sex	Source	Serology

Annex 1: Data collection instrument

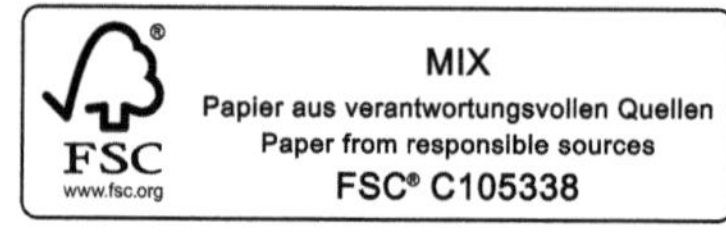

Printed by Books on Demand GmbH, Norderstedt / Germany